THE *Skinny*
SIRT
food diet

THE SKINNY SIRTFOOD DIET RECIPE BOOK
ACTIVATE YOUR 'SKINNY GENE'! CALORIE COUNTED SIRTFOOD RECIPES

ISBN 978-1-910771-90-7

A CIP catalogue record of this book is available from the British Library

• •

Disclaimer

Some recipes may contain nuts or traces of nuts. Those suffering from any allergies associated with nuts should avoid any recipes containing nuts or nut based oils. This information is provided and sold with the knowledge that the publisher and author do not offer any legal or other professional advice. In the case of a need for any such expertise consult with the appropriate professional. This book does not contain all information available on the subject, and other sources of recipes are available. This book has not been created to be specific to any individual's requirements. Before embarking on any diet seek advice from your doctor.

Every effort has been made to make this book as accurate as possible. However, there may be typographical and or content errors. Therefore, this book should serve only as a general guide and not as the ultimate source of subject information.

This book contains information that might be dated and is intended only to educate and entertain.
The author and publisher shall have no liability or responsibility to any person or entity regarding any loss or damage incurred, or alleged to have incurred, directly or indirectly, by the information contained in this book.

CONTENTS

DAY 6

DAY 7

SKINNY SIRTFOOD DIET PHASE 1 PLANNER: DAYS 4-7

SKINNY SIRTFOOD DIET PHASE 2: BREAKFAST RECIPES

SKINNY SIRTFOOD DIET PHASE 2: LUNCH RECIPES

SKINNY SIRTFOOD DIET PHASE 2: DINNER RECIPES 79

SKINNY SIRTFOOD DIET PHASE 2: SNACK & SAUCE RECIPES 97

OTHER COOKNATION TITLES 104

INTRODUCTION

The revolutionary Sirtfood diet for weight loss and health – it's about what you CAN eat not what you can't!

A diet that focuses on the positive effects of healthy balanced nutrition, works in perfect tandem with your body, can result in amazing weight loss (up to 7lbs in 7 days), increased energy levels, increased lean muscle, general heightened well being and rarely has you feeling hungry.

You will have likely read the headlines which have highlighted the inclusion and benefits of red wine, coffee and chocolate. Yes it's true they are all on the top 20 list of Sirt-rich foods and can definitely be enjoyed while still losing weight but there are so many other fantastic ingredients and health benefits to focus on when you follow the Sirtfood diet.

If your weight loss efforts in the past have focused on severe calorie restricted diets you'll no doubt be painfully aware that while they can indeed have dramatic slimming results they are also notoriously difficult to sustain. Prolonged calorie restriction/fasting even for two days of the week takes a lot of discipline and often leaves us feeling irritable, tired, hungry and generally miserable. Maintaining this type of diet long term is difficult and many of us fall off the wagon and inevitably end up back where we started often a pound or two heavier and even more demotivated.

So instead of fixating on the negative effects of a diet (e.g. all the foods you CAN'T eat), what if you could diet where the focus was on all the positive foods that you CAN and SHOULD be eating? That's got be good right? The psychological effect on this positive approach is huge in achieving your goals but more than that wouldn't you rather focus on the quality of your food rather than the quantity?

Step forward the Sirtfood Diet. A revolutionary new approach to health and weight loss which has come to the fore thanks to new scientific research which has identified turbocharging foods that activate the 'skinny gene' in all of us.

The science of the Sirtfood diet is fully explained by Aidan Goggins and Glen Matten in their breakthrough book 'The Sirtfood Diet'. Here they trialed their theory based on scientific research on members of one of London's most exclusive health clubs with amazing success. Participants experienced on average 7lbs weight loss in 7 days with increases in lean muscle too. We highly recommend you read their book for a full understanding of the science and research.

To follow is an outline of the Sirtfood diet and how it works backed up with over 75 recipes to get you started on phase 1 and 2 of the plan then 'SIRTifying' your eating habits long term so you can sustain your new healthy weight and start on the road to a long term nutrient rich diet.

THE 'SKINNY' GENE

This rather unscientific term relates to a group of genes in our body called sirtuins. Put simply, sirtuins relate to the body's metabolism, insulin and cell repair. Activating these genes is the key to aiding weight loss, making us healthier and living longer.

Research tells us that that there are 2 principal ways to spark theses super genes:

1)   **by restricting calories and exercising**
2)   **by SIRT activators**

We know that restricting calories (a measurement of energy) and expending more energy than we consume (a calorie deficit) will occur in weight loss and this indeed is also part of phase 1 & 2 of the Sirtfood diet.

Q):   So how do we use Sirt activators?

A):   By consuming foods that contain a natural rich source of SIRT activators – also called Sirtfoods.

Sirtfoods activate Sirtuins (the 'skinny' genes) and get to work triggering the body to stop storing fat and instead get its energy, not from primarily glucose, but breaking down the fat stores.

There are seven Sirtuins in the body, named Sirt 1 to Sirt 7, which control metabolism, insulin levels and cell repair. Research continues on the function of these genes but it is known that their activation is a key factor in weight loss, improved health and anti-ageing.

Sirtuins also reduce levels of the hormone IGF-1 (Insulin-like Growth Factor) which is directly responsible for the ageing process. IGF-1 causes the body to grow and produce new cells. By consuming a Sirtfood rich diet, levels of IGF-1 decrease which makes our body focus more on repairing cells which is key to slowing down the ageing process.

WHAT ARE SIRTFOODS?

Sirtfoods are a group of foods rich in special nutrients called polyphenols that when eaten activate sirtuins in our body in the same was as fasting does prompting fat burning while also increasing muscle and levels of cell repair.

Sirtfoods are prevalent in the diets of those with some of the lowest levels of disease and obesity around the world (known as 'blue zones) notably the Kuna American Indians who favour Sirt-rich cocoa in their diet to Okinawa in Japan where a range of nutrient rich Sirtfoods make up much of their daily intake. The well-known Mediterranean diet also contains Sirt-rich food like extra virgin olive oil, nuts, berries, red wine and dates and is key to keeping obesity levels low.

THE TOP SIRTFOODS

There are many foods that contain the powerful sirtuin-activating effects but research has identified the following top foods as being some of the most nutrient rich:

Birds-eye chilli	Red grapes & red wine	Olives & Extra Virgin Olive Oil	Soy & Tofu
Onions	Ground tumeric	Citrus fruits	Dark chocolate & cocoa powder
Buckwheat	Kale	Matcha green tea	

By increasing our daily intake of sirtuin activating foods (Sirtfoods) we can experience all the benefits of the Sirtfood diet – weight loss, more energy, feeling better, maintaining or increasing muscle. Research has also shown that combining Sirt-activating foods with fasting helps regulate appetite in the brain meaning no hunger pangs.

As you can see, the majority of the list of Sirtfoods are all recognisable, easily obtainable and affordable. You really don't need to alter your shopping list all that much to make it Sirt-friendly.

You may be looking at the list of Sirtfoods and wondering how to make a tasty Sirt-rich meal – that's where we come in. Our recipes combine the nutrient packed Sirtfoods with lean protein, omega-rich fish, good carbs and plenty of fresh fruit and veg to create delicious healthy meals.

MEAL PLANS

Our recipes follow the recommendations set out in The Sirtfood Diet by Aiden Goggins and Glen Matten. These are:

Phase 1 (7 days)

Days 1-3
Restricted fasting (approx. 1000 calories)
- 3 x Sirt smoothies
- 1 x Sirt meal

Days 4-7
Moderate fasting (approx. 1500 calories)
- 2 x Sirt smoothies
- 2 x Sirt meals
- 1 x Sirt snack

Phase 2 (14 days)

Days 1-14
Maintenance (approx. 1500 calories)
- 3 x Sirtfood meals
- 1 x Sirt smoothie
- Plus Sirtfood snacks

The Sirt smoothie is a fantastic way to ingest the nutrient rich Sirtfoods into your body. They are very easy to make, taste great and super-charge your system with the high content of Sirt goodness we are looking for. Our Sirt smoothie recipe stays the same throughout the 3 week programme.

Phase 1 is known as the 'hyper success' phase and is where you will see your most notable weight loss (up to 7lbs in 7 days) although remember that you may also increase muscle so don't completely rely on the bathroom scales. Look in the mirror and use your clothes to follow the changes in your body.

We have developed an easy to follow planner that will offer a number of meal options (including vegetarian) for Phase 1. All recipes are calorie counted so you can keep track of your daily intake and all are single servings.

Phase 2 will underpin the transformation in Phase 1, introducing Sirtfoods into your diet on a daily basis and continuing to lose weight at a healthy pace.

Although Phase 2 of the Sirtfood diet and indeed adopting the Sirtfood approach long term is not focused on calorie counting, by showing the calories for each meal it will make it easier for you to balance out your own Sirt-based recipes as you move beyond the initial 3 week plan.

During phase 2 you should be eating approx. 1500 calories per day. You will find a large selection of calorie counted Sirt-rich meals which we have split into breakfast, lunch, dinner and snacks. This allows you the freedom to choose your own meal combinations.

Recipes for phase 2 serve 1 or serve 4 allowing you integrate the meals with your family and/or to make ahead and freeze for another day.

These recipes, and those in phase 1, form the basis of your future Sirt meal choices as you adopt a healthier way of eating. Remember that you are in charge of what you eat and the Sirtfood diet is about inclusion. If you feel you are hungry during phase 2 then allow yourself one of the Sirtfood snacks or a square or two of dark chocolate. A small glass of red wine on the odd evening might also help keep you motivated.

MORE SIRTUIN ACTIVATING FOODS

While we've listed the most prolific Sirt-rich foods available there are many others which also pack a good punch of Sirt nutrients and which we have incorporated into our recipes. Examples of just some of the additional sirtuin activating foods are listed opposite. We would encourage you to research and seek out as many additional sirtuin activating foods when preparing your own recipes or perhaps to use as a substitute where a top sirtfood ingredient might be missing in your store cupboard.

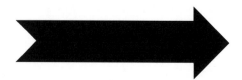

Blackberries	Spinach	Sardines	Coffee
Apples	Asparagus	Trout	Tea
Gogi berries	Cauliflower	Sardines	Fresh apple & orange juice
Blackcurrants	Parsley	Fresh tuna	Peppermint tea

SIRT PORTIONS

As time moves on you'll begin making up your own meals and create your own recipes as your Sirt journey continues beyond phase 2. As you do start to experiment with your own Sirt cooking it's helpful to know the quantity of each Sirtfood you should be using.

Take a look at the quantities of Sirt ingredients we use throughout the recipes in the book to guide you. Very broadly speaking a handful of the listed leaves, greens, veg and fruit constitutes a portion of Sirt food. A fruit juice or coffee portion is approximately 200ml/7floz, whilst dry spices would be approx. 1 teaspoon and fresh herbs 1 tablespoon.

ADVICE

- Try to consume your 3 juices evenly throughout the day and at least 30 minutes before a meal.

- Consume your last meal before 7pm. Out internal body clock knows when it's evening time and they process food less aggressively in the evening knowing that our bodies expend less energy. The result is more fat storage.

- Combine exercise throughout the 3 week plan. If you already exercise regularly continue as normal with your routine. If you are new to exercise avoid anything too rigorous during phase 1. Daily exercise combined with a Sirtfood diet will reap more health benefits.

- Use your appetite as guide. If you feel full when eating one of our meals don't feel you have to finish all of it. Remember that eating Sirtfoods while fasting means appetite is regulated to the brain so listen to your head as well as your stomach.

- Does following the Sirtfood diet mean I can drink more red wine and chocolate?
Unfortunately not! While red wine and 85% cocoa dark chocolate are both excellent Sirt-activating foods, everything should be in moderation. We would advise avoiding red wine (except in cooking) during phase 1 and then, if you choose, only a glass a day thereafter (no more than 5-6 small 175ml glasses per week according to the latest UK government guidelines on alcohol consumption). If in doubt abstain from alcohol altogether.

- Remember the Sirtfood diet is about inclusion. Focus on the amazing foods you should include in your diet and the many health benefits and don't focus on what you can't have.

· If you are pregnant or trying to conceive we do not recommend the Sirtfood diet.

· If you are currently taking any regular medication you should consult your doctor before starting any diet.

ABOUT

CookNation is the leading publisher of innovative and practical recipe books for the modern, health conscious cook.

CookNation titles bring together delicious, easy and practical recipes with their unique approach - easy and delicious, no-nonsense recipes - making cooking for diets and healthy eating fast, simple and fun.

With a range of #1 best-selling titles - from the innovative 'Skinny' calorie-counted series, to the 5:2 Diet Recipes collection - CookNation recipe books prove that 'Diet' can still mean 'Delicious'!

Visit **www.bellmackenzie.com** to browse the full catalogue.

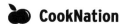 **CookNation**

THE *Skinny* SIRT
food diet

PHASE ① PLANNER
DAYS 1-3

DAY 1
3 x Sirt smoothies + 1 meal

Sirt Smoothie x 3 (p14)
+
Horseradish Flaked Salmon Fillet & Kale (p15)
or
Spiced Scrambled Omelette (V) (p16)
or
Stir-fried Peppers & Steak (p17)

DAY 2
3 x Sirt smoothies + 1 meal

Sirt Smoothie x 3 (p14)
+
Pak Choi & Prawns (p18)
or
Spiced Chicken & Brown Rice (p19)
or
Olive Caponata (V) (p20)

DAY 3
3 x Sirt smoothies + 1 meal

Sirt Smoothie x 3 (p14)
+
Cod & Olives With Buckwheat (p21)
or
Buckwheat Noodle Chicken Ramen (p22)
or
Coconut Milk Molee (V) (p23)

SIRT SMOOTHIE (V)

140 calories

PHASE 1 & 2

Ingredients

- 75g/3oz spinach
- 125g/4oz apple
- 50g/2oz strawberries
- 2 asparagus spears or 1 stalk of celery
- 1 tbsp lemon juice
- 1 tbsp flat leaf parsley
- Pinch of Matcha tea
- 3 tbsp water

Method

1 Rinse the spinach, apple & strawberries. Core and peel the apple. Remove any thick stalks from the asparagus or celery.. Chop the strawberries.

2 Add everything to the blender. Twist on the blade and blend until smooth. Add some more water if you want a thinner consistency.

CHEF'S NOTE
This Sirt staple should be used throughout Phase 1 & 2 of the Sirtfood diet.

HORSERADISH FLAKED SALMON FILLET & KALE

490 calories

DAY 1

Ingredients

- 200g/7oz skinless, boneless salmon fillet
- 50g/2oz green beans
- 75g/3oz kale
- 1 tbsp extra virgin olive oil
- ½ garlic clove, crushed
- 50g/2oz red onion, chopped
- 1 tbsp freshly chopped chives
- 1 tbsp freshly chopped flat leaf parsley
- 1 tbsp low fat crème fraiche
- 1 tbsp horseradish sauce
- 1 tsp lemon juice
- Salt & pepper to taste

Method

1 Season the salmon fillet and place under a preheated grill for 10-12 minutes or until cooked through. Flake and put to one side to cool.

2 Steam the kale & green beans for 5-10 minutes or until tender. Meanwhile heat the oil, garlic & chopped red onion in a saucepan and gently sauté for a few minutes. Add the steamed kale & greens beans. Stir well and cook for a minute or two longer.

3 In a seperate bowl gently combine together the chives, parsley, crème fraiche, horseradish sauce, lemon juice & cooled flaked salmon.

4 Heap the sautéed kale and beans onto a plate, sit the dressed salmon on top. Season & serve.

CHEF'S NOTE
Feel free to use pre-cooked salmon fillets if you are short of time.

SERVES 1

SPICED SCRAMBLED OMELETTE (V)

470 calories

DAY 1

Ingredients

- 100g/3½oz baby new potatoes, halved
- 125g/4oz tenderstem broccoli, roughly chopped
- 1 tbsp extra virgin olive oil
- 50g/2oz red onion, chopped
- ½ birds eye chilli, finely chopped

- 1-2 tsp turmeric
- 3 medium free-range eggs
- 1 tbsp freshly chopped flat leaf parsley
- 50g/2oz rocket
- Salt & pepper to taste

Method

1 Place the potatoes in boiling water. Boil for 5 minutes, add the broccoli and simmer for a few minutes longer or until the potatoes are tender. Drain and put to one side.

2 Meanwhile gently heat the olive oil in a frying pan and sauté the chopped red onion and chillies for a few minutes until softened. Add the potatoes, broccoli & turmeric to the pan and stir. Cook for a minute or two longer before adding the eggs.

3 Increase the heat. Keep moving everything quickly around the pan and cook until the eggs are scrambled. Check the seasoning, sprinkle the chopped parsley over the top & serve immediately with the rocket piled on the side of the plate.

CHEF'S NOTE
Protein-rich, this meal is bursting with Sirt goodness.

STIR-FRIED PEPPERS & STEAK

520 calories

DAY 1

Ingredients

- 125g/4oz sirloin steak
- 1 tbsp extra virgin olive oil
- 1 tsp paprika
- 50g/2oz red onion, chopped
- 1 garlic clove, crushed
- 1 red or yellow pepper, deseeded & sliced
- 50g/2oz red chicory/endive, chopped
- 100g/3½oz cherry tomatoes
- 50g/2oz celery, chopped
- 50g/2oz watercress
- 25g/1oz feta cheese, crumbled
- Salt & pepper to taste

Method

1 Trim any fat off the steak. Lightly brush with a little of the olive oil & all the paprika. Season and put a frying pan on a high heat.

2 In another pan gently sauté the red onions, garlic, peppers & chicory in the rest of the olive oil for 5-7 minutes or until tender.

3 Place the steak in the smoking hot dry pan and cook for 1-2 minutes each side, or to your liking. Leave to rest for 3 minutes and then finely slice.

4 Halve the tomatoes & combine with the watercress and celery. Tip the sauteed peppers and onions on top and sprinkle with the feta cheese.

5 Lay the sliced steak on top. Season and serve.

CHEF'S NOTE
Red chicory contains inulin which is a powerful probiotic.

PAK CHOI & PRAWNS

580 calories

DAY 2

Ingredients

- 75g/3oz brown rice
- 1 pak choi/bok choi, shredded
- 60ml/¼ cup chicken stock
- 1 tbsp extra virgin olive oil
- 1 garlic clove, crushed
- 50g/2oz red onion, chopped
- ½ birds eye chilli, finely chopped

- 1 tsp freshly grated ginger
- 125g/4oz shelled raw king prawns
- 1 tbsp soy sauce
- 1 tsp Chinese five spice powder
- 1 tbsp freshly chopped flat leaf parsley
- Salt & pepper to taste

Method

1 Place the brown rice in boiling water and cook until tender.

2 Meanwhile shred the pak choi and gently wilt in a frying pan with the chicken stock for a few minutes until tender.

3 Heat the olive oil in a frying pan and sauté the garlic, red onions, ginger and chillies for a minute or two.

4 Add the prawns, soy sauce & Chinese five spice powder & and cook until the prawns are pink.

5 When the prawns are cooked through. Add the drained brown rice to the pan and combine for a minute or two. Quickly toss through the wilted pak choi. Sprinkle the chopped parlsey over the top, season and serve immediately.

CHEF'S NOTE

Soy sauce is good source of daidzein and formononetin both known for their antioxidant properties.

SPICED CHICKEN & BROWN RICE

590 calories

DAY 2

Ingredients

- 75g/3oz brown rice
- 1 tbsp extra virgin olive oil
- 1 garlic clove, crushed
- 50g/2oz red onion, chopped
- ½ birds eye red chilli, deseeded & finely chopped
- 1 tsp turmeric
- ½ tsp ground coriander/cilantro
- 100g/3½oz skinless chicken breast, sliced
- 1 tbsp soy sauce
- 1 medium free-range egg
- 50g/2oz watercress
- Salt & pepper to taste

Method

1 Place the brown rice in boiling water and cook until tender.

2 Heat the olive oil in a frying pan and gently sauté the garlic, red onion and chilli for a minute or two.

3 Keep the contents of the pan moving around and add the turmeric, coriander, sliced chicken & soy sauce. Cook for 5-8 minutes or until the chicken is cooked through.

4 Add the drained rice to the pan along with the egg. Increase the heat, stir-fry for 3-4 minutes adding the watercress for the last 60 seconds..

5 Pile everything into a shallow bowl, season & serve.

CHEF'S NOTE
A garnish of freshly chopped flat leaf parsley and chives will give this dish an additional SIRT boost.

OLIVE CAPONATA (V)

520 calories

Ingredients

- 1 tbsp extra virgin olive oil
- 75g/3oz aubergine/egg plant, cubed
- 75g/3oz courgettes/zucchini, chopped
- 1 tsp dried oregano
- 50g/2oz red onion, chopped
- 50g/2oz celery, chopped
- 50g/2oz green beans, chopped
- 1 garlic clove, crushed

- 1 tbsp balsamic vinegar
- 1 tbsp capers, chopped
- 200g/7oz ripe plum tomatoes, roughly chopped
- 75g/3oz pitted black olives, sliced
- 1 tbsp sultanas, roughly chopped
- 125g/4oz cooked puy lentils
- Salt & pepper to taste

Method

1 Gently sauté the aubergines, courgettes, oregano, onions, celery, green beans and garlic in the olive oil for a few minutes until softened.

2 Add the balsamic vinegar, capers, tomatoes, olives & sultanas and continue to cook for 20-25 minutes or until everything is cooked through and tender.

3 Stir though the puy lentils, combine well, season & serve.

CHEF'S NOTE
Ready cooked Puy lentils are now widely available and cut down on cooking time.

COD & OLIVES WITH BUCKWHEAT

540 calories

DAY 3

Ingredients

- 1 tbsp extra virgin olive oil
- 75g/3oz white onion, chopped
- ½ birds eye red chilli, deseeded & finely chopped
- 1 garlic clove, crushed
- 200g/7oz ripe plum tomatoes, roughly chopped

- 1 tbsp sundried tomato puree
- 50g/2oz pitted black olives, sliced
- 150g/5oz skinless, boneless cod fillet
- 100g/3½oz buckwheat
- 1-2 tsp lemon juice
- 2 tbsp freshly chopped flat leaf parsley
- Salt & pepper to taste

Method

1 Gently sauté the onion, chilli and garlic in the olive oil for a few minutes until softened. Add the chopped tomatoes, puree & olives and leave to gently simmer for 10 minutes stirring occasionally.

2 Season the fish fillet, cut into thick slices, add to pan and combine well. Cover and leave to gently simmer for 10-15 minutes or until the fish is cooked through and piping hot.

3 Whilst the fish is cooking. Rinse the buckwheat and put in a saucepan with twice its volume of water. Bring to a simmer, cover tightly and reduce the heat to very low. Simmer for 10 minutes, or until all the water has been absorbed. Taste and add a splash more water and cook for a little longer if necessary.

4 Pile the buckwheat into a shallow bowl, combine with the lemon juice and fluff with a fork.

5 Tip the cod & sauce over the top, sprinkle with chopped parsley and serve.

CHEF'S NOTE
Unconnected to wheat, buckwheat is actually a relative of the rhubarb family.

21

BUCKWHEAT NOODLE CHICKEN RAMEN

SERVES 1

DAY 3

510 calories

Ingredients

- 50g/2oz leeks, sliced
- 50g/2oz celery, chopped
- 50g/2oz carrots, chopped
- 50g/2oz red chicory/endive, shredded
- 50g/2oz pak choi/bok choi, shredded
- 1 tsp dried thyme
- 500ml/2 cups chicken stock
- 75g/3oz cooked chicken breast, shredded
- 100g/3½oz tinned sweetcorn, drained
- 1 tbsp soy sauce
- 75g/3oz buckwheat (soba) noodles
- 1 bunch spring onions, sliced thinly lengthways
- 1 tbsp freshly chopped flat leaf parsley
- Salt & pepper to taste

Method

1 Place the leeks, celery & carrots in a saucepan along with the thyme and stock. Bring to the boil and simmer for 7-10 minutes or until all the vegetables are soft.

2 Place the contents of the pan into a blender. Blend to a smooth consistency and return to the pan.

3 Add the chicory, pak choi, shredded chicken, sweetcorn & noodles and cook for a further 6-8 minutes or until the ramen is piping hot and the noodles are tender.

4 Check the seasoning and serve with the sliced spring onions and parsley on top.

CHEF'S NOTE
Soba noodles are thin noodles made from buckwheat whereas udon noodles are made from wheat flour.

COCONUT MILK MOLEE (V)

540 calories

Ingredients

- 50g/2oz brown rice
- 1 garlic clove, crushed
- 50g/2oz red onion, chopped
- 1 tbsp extra virgin olive oil
- 50g/2oz soya beans
- 1 tbsp tomato puree

- 1 tsp each turmeric, cumin & coriander/cilantro
- 120ml/½ cup low fat coconut milk
- 3 medium free-range hard-boiled eggs
- 1 tbsp freshly chopped flat leaf parsley
- Salt & pepper to taste

Method

1 Place the brown rice in a pan of boiling water and cook until tender.

2 Gently sauté the garlic, red onion & soya beans in the olive oil for a few minutes until softened.

3 Stir through the tomato puree, dried spices & coconut milk until combined. Cut the eggs in half and place yolk side up, in the coconut milk. Gently cook until warmed through.

4 When everything is piping hot, drain the rice and spoon the curry on top.

5 Season and serve with parsley sprinkled over the top.

CHEF'S NOTE

While molee is traditionally a fish-based dish this is a great vegetarian alternative.

THE *Skinny* SIRT
food diet

PHASE ① PLANNER
DAYS 4-7

The planner has been put together to simplify meal times but feel free to choose any 2 meals of the 4 listed for each day

DAY 4

2 x Sirt smoothies + 2 meals + snack

Sirt Smoothie x 2 (p14)
+
Buckwheat Berry Breakfast Pancakes (V) (p26)
or
Fruity Green Breakfast Salad (V) (p27)
+
Steamed Salmon Soya Bean Salad (p28)
or
Chicken & Fried Cauliflower 'Rice' (p29)
+
Sweet Nut & Seed Snack (V) (p30)

DAY 5

2 x Sirt smoothies + 2 meals + snack

Sirt Smoothie x 2 (p14)
+
Indian Spiced Breakfast (V) (p31)
or
Energy Release Fruit Muesli (V) (p32)
+
Brown Rice & Italian Beans (V) (p33)
or
Chicken & Buckwheat Noodle Salad (p34)
+
Sweet Soy Edamame (V) (p35)

DAY 6

2 x Sirt smoothies + 2 meals + snack

Sirt Smoothie x 2 (p14)
+
Honey & Cinnamon Sirt Museli (V) (p36)
or
Fruit & Walnut Salad (V) (p37)
+
Pan Fried Tuna & Soya Beans (p38)
or
Nuoc Mam Cham (p39)
+
4 squares (40g) dark chocolate (85% cocoa)

DAY 7

2 x Sirt smoothies + 2 meals + snack

Sirt Smoothie x 2 (p14)
+
Pomegranate Quinoa (V) (p40)
or
Seabass With Caper & Parsley Mayonnaise (p41)
+
Turkey Curry & Cauliflower Rice (p42)
or
Soya Bean & Oregano Pasta (V) (p43)
+
Roasted Garlic Kale Chips (V) (p44)

BUCKWHEAT BERRY BREAKFAST PANCAKES (V)

430 calories

DAY 4

Ingredients

- 50g/2oz buckwheat flour
- 1 tbsp porridge oats
- 1 large free-range egg
- 120ml/½ cup milk
- 2 tsp honey

- 2 tsp extra virgin olive oil
- ½ tsp vanilla extract
- 50g/2oz blueberries
- 50g/2oz strawberries, sliced

Method

1 Add the flour, oats, egg, milk & honey to a blender. Pulse for a few seconds until you have a smooth batter.

2 Heat up a large frying pan and add the oil.

3 Make sure the oil properly covers the base of the pan, and when it's hot enough pour a quarter of the pancake batter in.

4 Gently cook for a minute or two. Flip it and cook for 30-60 seconds longer or until it's cooked through. Do the same with the rest of the mixture so that you end up with a stack of four pancakes.

5 Pile the fruit on top and serve.

CHEF'S NOTE

You can make more than one pancake at a time if your pan is large enough.

FRUITY GREEN BREAKFAST SALAD (V)

450 calories

DAY 4

Ingredients

- 75g/3oz avocado flesh, cubed
- 125g/5oz mango flesh, peeled, stoned & cubed
- 50g/2oz medjool dates, stoned and chopped
- 2 tsp extra virgin olive oil
- 75g/3oz vine ripened tomatoes, diced
- ½ tsp paprika
- ¼ birds eye chilli, deseeded & finely chopped
- 1 tbsp lime juice
- 1 tbsp freshly chopped flat leaf parsley
- 50g/2oz watercress
- Salt & pepper to taste

Method

1 Combine the cubed avocado, mango, dates, olive oil, tomatoes, paprika, chilli, lime & parsley together.

2 Allow to sit for a few minutes to let the flavour infuse.

3 Pile onto a bed of watercress, season & serve.

CHEF'S NOTE
Dates are a good source of the sirtuin-activating nutrients gallic & caffeic acid.

STEAMED SALMON SOYA BEAN SALAD

490 calories

DAY 4

Ingredients

- 150g/5oz skinless salmon fillet
- 1 tbsp soy sauce
- 1 tbsp lime juice
- 200g/7oz tenderstem broccoli, roughly chopped
- 50g/2oz soya beans
- ½ cucumber, diced
- ½ red pepper, deseeded & sliced
- 50g/2oz red onion, finely sliced
- 2 tsp olive oil
- 1 tbsp freshly chopped flat leaf parsley
- 1 tsp sesame seeds
- Salt & pepper to taste

Method

1 Season the salmon and brush with the soy sauce and lime juice. Place in the bottom tier of a steamer. Cover with the lid and leave to steam for 5 minutes.

2 Add the broccoli and soya beans to the second tier of the steamer, replace the lid and steam for another 4 minutes or until the fish is cooked through.

3 Take the veg out of the steamer and rinse under cold water for a second so that it stops cooking – you don't want it too soft.

4 Dry the veg off and tip into a bowl. Flake the salmon over the top. Combine the cucumber, peppers, red onion, olive oil & parsley together and add to the bowl. Sprinkle with sesame seeds and serve.

CHEF'S NOTE
This is ideal to prepare ahead for a nutrient rich packed-lunch.

CHICKEN & FRIED CAULIFLOWER 'RICE'

490 calories

DAY 4

Ingredients

- 250g/9oz cauliflower florets
- 2 tsp olive oil
- 50g/2oz red onion, chopped
- 1 garlic clove, crushed
- 1 tsp freshly grated ginger
- ½ red pepper, chopped & deseeded
- 1-2 tbsp soy sauce

- 1 large free-range egg
- 50g/2oz soya beans
- 125g/4oz cooked chicken breast, shredded
- 2 spring onions/scallions, chopped
- 2 tbsp freshly chopped chives
- Salt & pepper to taste

Method

1 Place the cauliflower florets in a food processor and pulse a few times until the cauliflower is the size of rice grains.

2 Place the 'rice' in a microwavable dish, cover and cook on full power for about 2 minutes or until it's piping hot. When it's done put to one side.

3 Whilst the rice is cooking heat the oil in a frying pan and sauté the onion, garlic, ginger & peppers for a few minutes. Add the chicken, soy sauce & soya beans to the pan and cook for a few minutes longer.

4 Add the 'rice' to the pan along with the soy sauce and move around well. Break the egg into the centre and quickly stir-fry until you see the egg 'set'.

5 Tip into a bowl and sprinkle the chopped spring onions and chives over the top.

CHEF'S NOTE
Add some finely chopped birds-eye chillies if you want some spice and additional luteolin (a flavonoid known for its anti-inflammatory properties).

SWEET NUT & SEED SNACK (V)

240 calories

DAY 4

Ingredients

- 75g/3oz pumpkin seeds
- 75g/3oz walnuts
- 1 tsp turmeric
- ½ tsp paprika

- 1 tsp sea salt flakes
- 1 tsp honey
- 1 tbsp extra virgin olive oil

Method

1 Preheat the oven to 180C/350F/Gas Mark 4.

2 Place all the ingredients into a large bowl and toss.

3 Combine everything really well and spread in a single layer on a baking sheet.

4 Bake in the oven for 12-15 minutes or until they are golden brown.

CHEF'S NOTE

Increase the honey if you like a particularly sweet snack.

INDIAN SPICED BREAKFAST (V)

425 calories

DAY 5

Ingredients

- 125g/4oz salad potatoes
- 2 medium free range eggs
- 1 tbsp extra virgin olive oil
- ¼ birds eye chilli, deseeded & finely chopped
- 50g/2oz red onion, sliced
- 50g/2oz kale, finely chopped
- 50g/2oz celery, sliced
- 1 tsp turmeric
- ½ tsp cumin
- Salt & pepper to taste

Method

1 Chop the potatoes into quarters and place in boiling water. Simmer for 5 and add the kale. Cook for a few minutes longer or until the potatoes are tender.

2 Meanwhile break the eggs into a bowl and lightly beat with a fork.

3 Heat the oil in a frying pan and gently sauté the onions and chilli for a few minutes until softened. Add the celery, turmeric & cumin and move around the pan.

4 Drain the potatoes and kale and add to the frying pan. Combine well and tip in the eggs. Increase the heat and cook until the eggs are scrambled.

5 Check the seasoning & serve immediately.

CHEF'S NOTE
Feel free to alter the amount of chilli to suit you own taste.

ENERGY RELEASE FRUIT MUESLI (V)

489 calories

DAY 5

Ingredients

- 100g/3½oz strawberries
- 100g/3½oz blueberries
- 50g/2oz apple
- 50g/2oz buckwheat flakes
- 50g/2oz medjool dates
- 1 tsp cocoa powder
- 100g/3½oz fat free Greek yoghurt

Method

1 Rinse the fruit well.

2 Slice the strawberries, core the apple and chop. Make sure the dates are stoned and chop these finely.

3 Combine everything together and serve immediately.

CHEF'S NOTE
Buckwheat flakes are available in most health food shops.

BROWN RICE & ITALIAN BEANS (V)

470 calories

DAY 5

Ingredients

- 50g/2oz brown rice
- 1 garlic clove
- 1 tbsp extra virgin olive oil
- 50g/2oz red onion
- 50g/2oz cherry tomatoes
- 1 tbsp flat leaf parsley, chopped
- 1 tbsp chives, chopped
- ½ birds eye chilli, deseeded & finely chopped

- 1 tsp freshly grated ginger
- 1 tbsp lime juice
- 50g/2oz cucumber
- 150g/5oz tinned cannellini or haricot beans, drained
- 50g/2oz celery sliced
- Salt & pepper to taste

Method

1 Place the brown rice in boiling water and cook until tender. Drain and set to one side.

2 Meanwhile put all the other ingredients, except the beans and celery, in the food processor and pulse until everything is chopped up. Don't turn it into a puree, just pulse a couple of times to make a chunky dressing.

3 When the rice is ready tip into a bowl and fluff it up with a fork. Add the chunky dressing from the food processor and combine really well, along with the drained beans.

4 Check the seasoning and serve.

CHEF'S NOTE
This is a great make-ahead recipe for a workday lunch or when you are on-the-go.

CHICKEN & BUCKWHEAT NOODLE SALAD

529 calories

DAY 5

Ingredients

- 50g/2oz buckwheat noodles
- ½ vegetable stock cube
- 50g/2oz cucumber
- 50g/2oz red chicory/endive
- 50g/2oz red onion
- 4 spring onions/scallions
- 150g/5oz cooked chicken breast, shredded
- ½ birds eye chilli, deseeded & finely chopped
- 2 tsp sesame oil
- 2 tsp soy sauce
- 2 tbsp flat leaf parsley, chopped
- 1 tbsp fresh coriander, chopped
- 1 tbsp chopped peanuts
- Salt & pepper to taste

Method

1 Crumble the stock cube in a pan of boiling water and stir to dissolve. Add the noodles, cover and leave to cook on the hob for a few minutes while you make the rest of the salad.

2 Cube up the cucumber and thinly slice the chicory, red onion and spring onions. Throw these in a bowl with the shredded chicken and chilli.

3 Drain the noodles, rinse in cold water and quickly stir through the sesame oil and soy sauce. Toss the noodles and fresh herbs with the chicken and onions.

4 Sprinkle with the chopped peanuts and eat straight away.

CHEF'S NOTE
Use prawns instead of chicken if you prefer.

SWEET SOY EDAMAME (V)

207 calories

DAY 5

Ingredients

- 200g/7oz edamame (soya beans still in their pods)
- 1 tbsp honey
- 2 tbsp soy sauce
- 2 tbsp water
- 1 tsp extra virgin olive oil

Method

1 Add the edamame to a pan of boiling water and simmer for 4 minutes. Drain and pat dry.

2 Meanwhile heat a saucepan with the honey, soy sauce, water and oil. Simmer for a few minutes until the sauce begins to thicken slightly (make sure you don't burn the honey).

3 Toss the edamame in and combine well. Delicious as a warm or cold snack.

CHEF'S NOTE
Try making a large batch of the sweet soy dressing so that you can make this easy snack anytime you like.

HONEY & CINNAMON SIRT MUSELI (V)

457 calories

DAY 6

Ingredients

- 100g/3½oz strawberries
- 100g/3½oz apple
- 25g/1oz walnuts,
- 50g/2oz buckwheat flakes
- 2 tsp honey
- 100g/3½oz fat free Greek yoghurt
- ½ tsp ground cinnamon

Method

1 Rinse the fruit well.

2 Slice the strawberries, core & chop the apple. Finely chop the walnuts.

3 Combine everything together and serve immediately,

CHEF'S NOTE
You could add some desiccated coconut to this muesli too.

FRUIT & WALNUT SALAD (V)

453 calories

DAY 6

Ingredients

- 125g/4oz orange (1 medium orange)
- 75g/3oz strawberries
- 6 black olives
- 1 tbsp extra virgin olive oil
- 2 tsp red wine vinegar
- 50g/2oz watercress

- 6 walnuts halves, chopped
- 2 tbsp flat leaf parsley, chopped
- Handful of young lovage leaves
- 50g/2oz feta cheese
- Salt & pepper to taste

Method

1 Remove the peel and pith from the orange and separate into segments. Slice each of these segments into 3 pieces.

2 Slice the strawberries and olives. Combine these, along with the orange pieces, with the olive oil and red wine vinegar.

3 Place the watercress in a shallow bowl and sit the dressed fruit on top. Sprinkle with the walnuts, parsley and lovage leaves.

4 Crumble the feta cheese over the top and serve.

CHEF'S NOTE
If you can't source lovage use additional flat leaf parsley.

PAN FRIED TUNA & SOYA BEANS

540 calories

DAY 6

Ingredients

- 1 tbsp soy sauce
- 1 tsp freshly grated ginger
- 2 spring onions/scallions, finely chopped
- 1 tbsp extra virgin olive oil
- 175g/6oz fresh tuna fillet weighing

- 1 pak choi/bok choi, quartered
- 50g/2oz soya beans
- 1 tbsp balsamic vinegar
- 50g/2oz watercress
- Salt & pepper to taste

Method

1 First make a dressing by mixing together the soy sauce, ginger & finely chopped spring onions.

2 Place a frying pan on a medium/high heat with the olive oil. Season the tuna fillet and add to the pan along with the pak choi and soya beans. Pour the balsamic vinegar over the top of the fillet and cook the tuna for 2 minutes each side. (Keep the vegetables moving around the pan, adding a splash of water if you need to).

3 Remove the tuna from the pan and leave to rest but carry on cooking the veg for a minute or two longer.

4 Thinly slice the tuna and arrange on a plate with the pak choi, soya beans and watercress on the side. Drizzle the soy sauce dressing all over the tuna slices and serve.

CHEF'S NOTE

Reduce the cooking time if you prefer your tuna rare.

NUOC MAM CHAM

520 calories

DAY 6

Ingredients

- 50g/2oz brown rice
- 1 tbsp extra virgin olive oil
- 50g/2oz red onion
- 50g/2oz green beans, chopped
- 2 garlic cloves, crushed
- 1 birds eye chilli, finely chopped (leave the seeds in)
- 2 tbsp lime juice
- 2 tbsp fish sauce
- 2 tsp caster sugar
- 75g/3oz cooked chicken breast, shredded
- 1 tbsp flat leaf parsley, chopped
- 50g/2oz rocket
- Salt & pepper to taste

Method

1 Cook the rice in boiling water until tender and drain.

2 Meanwhile heat up a frying pan with the olive oil and start sautéing the onions for a few minutes until softened

3 While the onions are cooking combine the garlic cloves, chilli, lime juice, fish sauce and caster sugar to make a spicy, sweet & sour dressing.

4 Tip the drained rice and shredded chicken into the pan with the onions and warm for a few minutes until everything is piping hot. Add the rocket for the last 60 seconds until it is gently wilted.

5 Load the chicken & rice into a bowl, drizzle the spicy dressing over the top and sprinkle with parsley.

CHEF'S NOTE
Balance the chilli, lime and sugar to suit your own taste in the fiery dressing.

POMEGRANATE QUINOA (V)

430 calories

······· *Ingredients* ·······

- 75g/3oz quinoa
- 250ml/1 cup hot vegetable stock
- 1 whole pomegranate
- 2 tsp lemon juice
- 1 tbsp extra virgin olive oil
- 1 tbsp fresh mint, chopped
- 2 tbsp flat leaf parsley, chopped
- 50g/2oz carrot, grated
- 50g/2oz celery, sliced
- Salt & pepper to taste

······· *Method* ·······

1 Put the quinoa and stock in a saucepan, cover and cook for about 20 minutes or until it's tender. (Add more stock if you need to and when it's ready drain off any excess liquid).

2 While the quinoa is cooking get the seeds out of the pomegranate. To do this just cut the fruit in half, place face down on a chopping board and bang the back of each halve hard with a spoon. The seeds should come shooting out, pick out any that are left in the rind.

3 Once the quinoa is ready fluff it up with a fork and combine it with the pomegranate seeds, lemon juice, olive oil, mint and parsley. Pile the grated carrot and sliced celery on top. Season and serve.

CHEF'S NOTE
Originally native to Persia pomegranates are rich in vitamins C & D.

SOYA BEAN & OREGANO PASTA (V)

480 calories

DAY 7

Ingredients

- 75g/3oz shelled fresh soya beans
- 1 tbsp extra virgin olive oil
- 6 anchovy fillets, drained
- 2 garlic cloves, crushed
- 75g/3oz red onion, sliced
- 75g/3oz ripe plum tomatoes, roughly chopped
- 2 tsp dried oregano
- 75g/3oz buckwheat pasta
- Salt & pepper to taste

Method

1 Place the soya beans in a pan of boiling water, cook for 2 minutes and drain.

2 Meanwhile heat the olive oil in a high-sided frying pan and gently sauté the anchovy fillets, garlic, red onions, chopped tomatoes, soya beans and oregano whilst you put the penne on to cook in a pan of boiling water.

3 When the penne is cooked, drain and add to the frying pan. Toss well, season and serve.

CHEF'S NOTE
Use whichever shaped buckwheat pasta you have to hand.

SEA BASS WITH CAPER & PARSLEY MAYONNAISE

490 calories

DAY 7

Ingredients

- 1 tbsp extra virgin olive oil
- 75g/3oz white onion, chopped
- 1 garlic clove, crushed
- 200g/7oz sea bass fillet
- 50g/2oz red chicory/endive, chopped
- 125g/4oz cherry tomatoes, halved
- 50g/2oz celery sliced

- 1 tbsp mayonnaise
- 1 tbsp capers, rinsed & chopped
- 1 tsp lemon juice
- 1 tbsp flat leaf parsley, chopped
- 50g/2oz rocket
- Salt & pepper to taste

Method

1 Place a frying pan on a medium heat with the olive oil and sauté the onions & garlic for a few minutes until softened.

2 Season the sea bass fillet and add to the pan along with the chicory, tomatoes and celery. Fry for about 6 minutes or until the fish is cooked through (turn the fish after 3 minutes).

3 Meanwhile combine the mayonnaise, capers, lemon juice and parsley together.

4 Remove everything from the pan piece by piece and arrange on the plate with the rocket and caper mayonnaise.

CHEF'S NOTE
The sea bass may need less/more time depending on how thick the fillet is.

TURKEY CURRY & CAULIFLOWER RICE

SERVES 1

DAY 7

540 calories

Ingredients

- 50g/2oz red onion, chopped
- 75g/3oz kale, chopped
- 1 garlic clove, crushed
- 1 tbsp extra virgin olive oil
- 125g/4oz cherry tomatoes, chopped
- 25g/1oz medjool dates, finely chopped
- 125g/4oz turkey breast, sliced

- 2 tsp medium curry powder
- 1 tsp turmeric
- 2 tbsp coconut cream
- 2 tbsp flat leaf parsley, chopped
- 200g/7oz cauliflower florets
- Salt & pepper to taste

Method

1 Get the onions, kale, garlic, cherry tomatoes & dates gently cooking in a frying pan with the olive oil. Sauté for a few minutes and then add the turkey, curry powder & turmeric (add a little more olive oil if needed).

2 Stir-fry for a few minutes until the turkey is cooked then stir through the coconut cream and parsley.

3 Meanwhile place the cauliflower florets in a food processor and pulse a few times until the cauliflower is the size of rice grains.

4 Place the 'rice' in a microwavable dish, cover and cook on full power for about 2 minutes or until it's piping hot.

5 Tip the 'rice' into a shallow bowl and pour the curry over the top.

CHEF'S NOTE
Medjool dates take the place of sultanas in this traditional Asian dish.

43

ROASTED GARLIC KALE CHIPS (V)

190 calories

DAY 7

Ingredients

- 200g/7oz kale
- 1-2 tsp sea salt flakes
- 2 tbsp extra virgin olive oil
- 1 garlic clove, crushed

Method

1 Preheat the oven to 180C/350F/Gas Mark 4.

2 Remove the thick stalks from the kale and tear the leaves into small bite size pieces.

3 Place these in a large bowl along with the salt, oil and garlic cloves.

4 Combine everything well and spread in a single layer on a baking sheet.

5 Bake in the oven for 12-15 minutes or until the edges begin to brown but are not burnt.

CHEF'S NOTE
This is a great snack to keep to hand throughout the day if you feel your energy levels dropping.

THE *Skinny*
SIRT
f o o d d i e t

PHASE ②PLANNER
DAYS 1-14

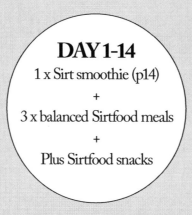

DAY 1-14
1 x Sirt smoothie (p14)
+
3 x balanced Sirtfood meals
+
Plus Sirtfood snacks

Phase 2 lasts for 14 days.

Unlike phase 1 where we provided a detailed daily planner, for phase 2 you are free to choose any meal combination from phase 2 breakfast, lunch and dinner recipes.

Whilst not too much emphasis should be put on calorie counting, for the sake of knowing your intake, you should aim for around 1500 calories each day for phase 2.

Each recipe is Sirt-rich and calorie counted so you can chose which meals work best for you on any given day.

You can also top up with one of the delicious sirt snacks.

For the next 14 days you should eat 3 meals per day, 1 Sirt smoothie and a snack if appropriate.

Recipes for phase 2 serve 1 or 4 allowing you to integrate the meals with your family and/or to make ahead and freeze for another day.

These recipes, and those in phase 1, form the basis of your future Sirt meal choices as you adopt a healthier way of eating. Remember that you are in charge of what you eat and the Sirtfood diet is about inclusion. If you feel you are hungry during phase 2 then allow yourself one of the Sirtfood snacks or a square or two of dark chocolate. A small glass of red wine on the odd evening might also help keep you motivated.

THE *Skinny* SIRT food diet

PHASE ②
BREAKFAST RECIPES
FOLLOW FOR 14 DAYS

BUCKWHEAT & BLUEBERRY PANCAKE STACK (V)

450 calories

Ingredients

- 120ml/½ cup milk
- 1 medium free-range egg
- Pinch of salt
- 50g/2oz buckwheat flour
- 50g/2oz blueberries
- 2 tsp extra virgin olive oil
- 1 tbsp maple syrup

Method

1 Beat together the milk, egg and salt.

2 Place the buckwheat in another bowl.

3 Gradually add milk mixture to the flour and stir until you get a smooth batter. Add the blueberries.

4 Add a little of the oil to a hot pan, pour in a quarter of the mixture and cook for 1-2 minutes or until golden on each side.

5 Remove from the pan and place to one side while you cook the others.

6 Serve with maple syrup drizzled over the top.

CHEF'S NOTE
Keep the pancakes warm while you cook your stack.

HOT SCRAMBLED EGGS (V)

307 calories

Ingredients

- 1 tbsp extra virgin olive oil
- 50g/2oz shallots, chopped
- ½ bird's-eye chilli, finely chopped
- 1 tsp turmeric
- 1 tsp ground coriander/cilantro

- 2 medium free-range eggs
- 2 tbsp freshly chopped flat leaf parsley
- 50g/2oz rocket
- Salt & pepper to taste

Method

1 Gently heat the olive oil in a frying pan and sauté the chopped shallots and chillies for a few minutes until softened.

2 Add the eggs, turmeric, coriander and fresh parsley to the pan. Increase the heat. Keep moving everything quickly around the pan and cook until the eggs are scrambled.

3 Check the seasoning and serve immediately with the rocket piled on the side of the plate.

CHEF'S NOTE
You could add some chopped ham or bacon to these easy scrambled eggs.

MATCHA MORNING YOGHURT (V)

310 calories

Ingredients

- 180g/6oz fat-free Greek yogurt
- 1 tbsp honey
- 1 tsp Matcha green tea
- 6 walnut halves
- 100g/3½oz strawberries

Method

1 Place the yogurt, honey in the blender together with the coconut match tea.

2 Twist on the blade and pulse for a few seconds to combine. Tip into a bowl.

3 Meanwhile rinse the strawberries, remove the green tops and finely chop, along with the walnuts.

4 Sprinkle both onto the yogurt and serve.

CHEF'S NOTE
Use more or less honey to suit your own taste.

COCOA STRAWBERRY MILK (V)

175 calories

Ingredients

- 120ml/½ cup light coconut milk
- 100g/3½oz strawberries
- 50g/2oz kale
- 1 tbsp cocoa powder
- Ice

Method

1 Rinse the strawberries and remove the green tops. Rinse the kale and remove any thick stalks.

2 Place the strawberries and kale in the blender together with the coconut milk and cocoa powder. Add ice, but make sure it doesn't go past the MAX line on your machine.

3 Twist on the blade and blend until smooth.

CHEF'S NOTE
This sweet smoothie also makes a great mid-morning snack.

KALE, APPLE & GRAPE SMOOTHIE (V)

230 calories

········· *Ingredients* ·········

- 60g/2½oz kale
- 100g/3½oz apple
- 15 seedless red grapes

- 3 tbsp low-fat Greek yoghurt
- 25g/1oz chopped avocado
- 2 tsp fresh lime juice

········· *Method* ·········

1 Rinse the kale, apple and grapes. Core and peel the apple.

2 Peel and de-stone the avocado

3 Add everything to the blender. Twist on the blade and blend until smooth. Add some water if you want a thinner consistency.

CHEF'S NOTE
You could also add a small handful of parsley to this creamy smoothie.

PARSLEY & GINGER JUICE (V)

190 calories

Ingredients

- 125g/4oz apple
- 150g/5oz cucumber
- 75g/3oz kale
- 1 tsp grated ginger
- 2 tsp lemon juice
- 1 tbsp flat leaf parsley, chopped
- 1 tbsp pumpkin seeds
- Water

Method

1 Rinse the apple, cucumber and kale. Remove any thick stalks from the kale. Core, peel and roughly chop the apple. Chop the cucumber. Peel and grate the ginger.

2 Add everything to the blender. Twist on the blade and blend until smooth. Add some water if you want a thinner consistency.

CHEF'S NOTE
Make sure your blender can handle pumpkin seeds.

STRAWBERRY NUT SMOOTHIE (V)

330 calories

Ingredients

- 50g/2oz celery
- 125g/4oz strawberries
- 50g/2oz kale
- 120ml/4floz light coconut milk
- 25g/1oz walnuts

Method

1 Rinse the celery and chop. Rinse the strawberries and remove the green tops. Rinse the kale and remove any thick stalks.

2 Place these in the blender together with the coconut milk and walnuts.

3 Twist on the blade and blend until smooth.

CHEF'S NOTE
Add water or more coconut milk if you want to alter the consistency.

COCOA CINNAMON MOCHA (V)

199 calories

Ingredients

- 180ml/¾ cup cooled black coffee
- 50g/2oz kale
- 50g/2oz medjool dates
- 2 tbsp cocoa powder
- 60ml/½ cup unsweetened almond milk
- ¼ tsp ground cinnamon

Method

1 Rinse the kale and remove any thick stalks.

2 Chop the dates and place these in the blender together with all the other ingredients.

3 Twist on the blade and blend until smooth.

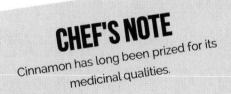

CHEF'S NOTE
Cinnamon has long been prized for its medicinal qualities.

GREEN ALMOND MILK SMOOTHIE (V)

310 calories

Ingredients

- 50g/2oz kale
- 50g/2oz watercress
- 2 tbsp flat leaf parsley, chopped
- 200g/7oz apple, peeled, cored & chopped
- 250ml/1 cup almond milk
- 100g/3½oz banana
- 50g/2oz pineapple
- Water

Method

1 Rinse the kale well and remove any thick stalks.

2 Peel the banana and break into three pieces.

3 Add all the ingredients the your smoothie maker/ blender.

4 Twist on the blade and blend until smooth.

CHEF'S NOTE

Kale is believed to help prevent cardiovascular disease, several types of cancer, asthma, rheumatoid arthritis, and pre-mature aging of the skin.

CREAMY MATCHA TEA ICE SMOOTHIE (V)

430 calories

Ingredients

- 50g/2oz kale
- 125g/4oz apple, peeled & cored
- 50g/2oz celery
- 125g/4oz avocado

- 1 medium banana, peeled
- 120ml/½ cup milk
- 1 tsp matcha tea powder
- A few ice cubes

Method

1 Rinse the kale, apple and celery. Core the apple and chop up along with the kale, celery, avocado and banana.

2 Add all the ingredients to the blender.

3 Twist on the blade and blend until smooth.

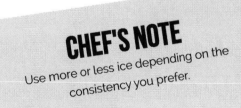

CHEF'S NOTE
Use more or less ice depending on the consistency you prefer.

STRAWBERRY SIRT SMOOTHIE (V)

430 calories

Ingredients

- 125g/4oz strawberries
- 25g/1oz kale
- 50g/2oz medjool dates
- 125g/4oz Greek yoghurt
- 120ml/½ cup soya milk
- 25g/1oz walnuts
- 1 tsp honey

Method

1 Rinse the strawberries & kale. Remove any thick stalks from the kale and make sure the dates are pitted.

2 Add all the ingredients to the blender.

3 Twist on the blade and blend until smooth.

CHEF'S NOTE
Almond milk works just as well in this smoothie too. Feel free to add more milk or yogurt to get the consistency right.

THE *Skinny*
SIRT
food diet

PHASE ②
LUNCH RECIPES
FOLLOW FOR 14 DAYS

BROCCOLI & CAULIFLOWER SOUP (V)

190 calories

Ingredients

- 1 tbsp extra virgin olive oil
- 75g/3oz shallots, chopped
- 600g/1lb 5oz cauliflower florets, chopped
- 200g/7oz broccoli florets, chopped
- 75g/3oz potatoes, peeled & chopped
- 1 tsp ground turmeric
- 1lt/4 cups vegetable stock/broth
- 250ml/1 cup milk
- 4 tbsp flat leaf parsley, finely chopped
- Salt & pepper to taste

Method

1 Gently sauté the shallots in the olive oil for a few minutes.

2 Add all the ingredients, except the milk and parsley, to a saucepan.

3 Bring to the boil and leave to simmer for 10-12 minutes or until the vegetables are tender.

4 Blend to a smooth consistency, add the milk, and heat through for a minute or two. Check the seasoning and serve with parsley sprinkled over the top.

CHEF'S NOTE
You could also add some finely chopped bird's-eye chillies as a spicy garnish for this soup.

ASPARAGUS SOUP (V)

218 calories

Ingredients

- 2 tbsp extra virgin olive oil
- 2 garlic cloves, crushed
- 1 leek, chopped
- 75g/3oz celery, sliced
- 75g/3oz shallots, sliced
- 200g/7oz fresh asparagus, trimmed and roughly chopped

- 4 tbsp flat leaf parsley, chopped
- 1lt/4 cups vegetable stock
- 125g/4oz buckwheat pasta
- 1 tbsp single cream
- Salt & pepper to taste

Method

1 Gently sauté the leek, celery, shallots and garlic in the olive oil for a few minutes.

2 Add all the other ingredients to the pan. Bring to the boil, cover and leave to simmer for 8-10 minutes or until the pasta is tender. Blend to your preferred consistency, season and serve with a little cream drizzled over the top.

CHEF'S NOTE
Break the buckwheat into very small pieces to make pasta soup-sized pieces.

CHICORY & RED ONION SALAD (V)

280 calories

Ingredients

- 125g/4oz vine ripened tomatoes
- 75g/3oz red onion
- 75g/3oz red chicory/endive
- 100g/3½oz baby spinach leaves
- 50g/2oz cooked soya beans
- 1 tbsp each freshly chopped basil, mint & flat leaf parsley
- 1 tbsp extra virgin olive oil
- 2 tsp balsamic vinegar
- Lemon wedges to serve
- Salt & pepper to taste

Method

1 First finely dice the tomatoes. Finely slice the red onion and chicory.

2 Toss together with the spinach leaves, soya beans chopped herbs, olive oil and balsamic.

3 Season to your taste and serve with lemon wedges.

CHEF'S NOTE

This is a very simple salad. If you are making ahead for a packed lunch don't toss in the oil or vinegar until you are ready to eat.

CHICKEN & KALE BUCKWHEAT PENNE

300 calories

Ingredients

- 200g/7oz skinless chicken breast, sliced
- 300g/11oz buckwheat penne pasta
- 1 tbsp extra virgin olive oil
- 2 garlic cloves, crushed
- 1 tsp dried oregano
- 200g/7oz kale, chopped
- 60ml/¼ cup chicken stock
- Salt & pepper to taste

Method

1 Heat the olive oil in a frying pan and begin cooking the sliced chicken for 3-4 minutes. Meanwhile cook the penne in a pan of boiling water until tender.

2 Add the garlic, oregano, kale & stock to the frying pan and cook until everything is tender and piping hot.

3 Drain the cooked penne and add to the frying pan.

4 Toss well, season and serve.

CHEF'S NOTE
Dried oregano is preferable to fresh oregano on the Sirt diet.

CAPER & DATE BUCKWHEAT SPAGHETTI (V)

420 calories

Ingredients

- 300g/11oz ripe cherry tomatoes
- 2 tbsp capers
- 75g/3oz medjool dates
- 300g/11oz buckwheat noodles/spaghetti
- 2 tbsp olive oil
- 1 garlic cloves, crushed
- 2 tbsp sundried tomato puree/paste
- 4 tbsp freshly chopped flat leaf parsley
- Salt & pepper to taste

Method

1 Half the cherry tomatoes and roughly chop the capers & dates.

2 Cook the pasta in a pan of water until tender.

3 Meanwhile heat the olive oil and gently sauté the garlic, cherry tomatoes, capers, dates and sundried tomato puree whilst the pasta cooks.

4 Drain the cooked pasta and add to the frying pan. Toss well and serve with chopped parsley on top.

CHEF'S NOTE

Feel free to serve with some watercress or rocket to increase your Sirt intake.

BLACK OLIVE & RED ONION BUCKWHEAT FUSILLI (V)

402 calories

Ingredients

- 1 tbsp balsamic vinegar
- 300g/11oz buckwheat fusilli
- 2 tbsp olive oil
- 1 garlic clove, crushed
- 50g/2oz red onion, sliced
- 300g/11oz ripe plum tomatoes
- 125g/4oz pitted black olives, sliced
- 50g/2oz kale, finely chopped
- 2 tbsp freshly chopped basil
- 2 tbsp flat leaf parsley, chopped
- Salt & pepper to taste

Method

1 Dice the ripe tomatoes and place in a bowl with the balsamic vinegar and some seasoning.

2 Cook the pasta in a pan of boiling water until tender.

3 Meanwhile heat the olive oil in a high-sided frying pan and gently sauté the garlic, red onion, tomatoes, olives and kale whilst the pasta cooks.

4 Drain the cooked pasta and add to the frying pan. Toss well, sprinkle with freshly chopped herbs, season & serve.

CHEF'S NOTE
Buckwheat pasta is readily available at most health foods stores.

EXTRA VIRGIN BUCKWHEAT SPAGHETTI (V)

395 calories

Ingredients

- 300g/11oz buckwheat noodles/spaghetti
- 3 tbsp extra virgin olive oil
- 3 garlic cloves, crushed
- 75g/3oz shallots, sliced
- 2 tbsp lemon juice
- 75g/3oz rocket
- 25g/1oz Parmesan shavings
- 4 tbsp freshly chopped flat leaf parsley
- Salt & pepper to taste

Method

1 Cook the buckwheat pasta in a pan of boiling water until tender.

2 Meanwhile heat the oil and gently sauté the garlic & shallots in a high sided frying pan whilst the pasta cooks.

3 Drain the cooked pasta and add to the frying pan. Toss well, add the rocket, sprinkle with freshly chopped parsley and Parmesan, season & serve.

CHEF'S NOTE
This is a simple Mediterranean recipe. Great for a quick and easy supper.

SWEET KALE & CARROT SOUP (V)

130 calories

Ingredients

- 150g/5oz kale
- 400g/14oz carrot
- 1 tbsp extra virgin olive oil
- 25g/1oz shallots, chopped
- 25g/1oz celery, chopped
- 1.25lt/5 cups vegetable stock/broth
- 1 tbsp honey
- 50g/2oz watercress, chopped
- Salt & pepper to taste

Method

1 Rinse and chop the kale & carrots (no need to peel).

2 Heat the oil in a saucepan and add the shallots & celery. Sauté for a minute or two before adding the stock, kale and carrots.

3 Turn up the heat, bring to the boil and simmer for 7-10 minutes or until all the vegetables are soft.

4 Add the honey and stir well.

5 Blend to a smooth consistency, check the seasoning and serve with the chopped watercress sitting on top.

CHEF'S NOTE
Remove any thick kale stalks before chopping the leaves.

FETA, APPLE & DATE SALAD (V)

460 calories

Ingredients

- 1 raw beetroot bulb, peeled
- 125g/4oz apple peeled & cored
- 50g/2oz medjool dates, stoned
- 1 tbsp freshly chopped oregano
- 1 tbsp balsamic vinegar

- 1 tbsp extra virgin olive oil
- 50g/2oz feta cheese
- 75g/4oz watercress
- Salt & pepper to taste

Method

1 Grate, or finely chop, the beetroot bulbs – ideally in a food processor.

2 Cut the apple into fine slices, chop the dates and gently combine both with the grated beetroot.

3 Add the oregano, balsamic vinegar & oil to the salad and mix well.

4 Check the seasoning and arrange on a bed of watercress with the feta cheese crumbled over the top.

CHEF'S NOTE
Use more or less balsamic vinegar to suit your own taste.

SALMON FILLET & SPRING GREENS

399 calories

Ingredients

- 150g/5oz skinless salmon fillet
- 150g/3oz savoy cabbage
- 75g/3oz soya beans
- 1 tbsp capers

- 1 tbsp fat free Greek yoghurt
- 1 tbsp horseradish sauce
- 1 tsp lemon juice
- Salt & pepper to taste

Method

1 Preheat the grill to a medium/high heat.

2 Season the salmon and cook under the grill for 4-6 minutes each side or until cooked through. Gently flake with a fork and put to one side to cool.

3 Plunge the cabbage and soya peas into a pan of boiling water and cook for 2 minutes.

4 Rinse and chop the capers. Mix together with the yoghurt, horseradish & lemon juice.

5 Gently combine the flaked salmon with the caper mayonnaise.

6 Drain the cabbage and beans. Toss with the salmon and caper mayonnaise. Season and serve.

CHEF'S NOTE
A top 20 Sirt food: capers are a good source of vitamin K, fibre and iron.

FRUITY CHICKEN COUSCOUS

394 calories

Ingredients

- 500ml/2 cups chicken stock
- 75g/3oz buckwheat
- 50g/2oz sultanas
- 150g/5oz cooked chicken breast
- 50g/2oz red onions, chopped
- 1 garlic clove, crushed
- 1 tsp ground coriander/cilantro
- 1 tbsp lemon juice
- Lemon wedges to serve
- 2 tbsp flat leaf parsley, chopped
- Salt & pepper to taste

Method

1 Simmer the buckwheat in the boiling stock for about 10 mins or until it's cooked through. Drain and put to one side.

2 Roughly chop the sultanas & chicken breast.

3 Gently sauté the chopped red onions, garlic, ground coriander & lemon juice for a few minutes.

4 Add the chicken and sultanas to warm through for a minute or two.

5 Fluff the buckwheat with a fork and pile into the onion pan. Mix well, season and serve with fresh lemon wedges on the side and chopped parsley sprinkled over the top.

CHEF'S NOTE
Fresh mint is also a good addition to this dish if you want to put your own twist on things.

PRAWN & CHICORY BEANS

395 calories

Ingredients

- 2 tbsp extra virgin olive oil
- 75g/3oz shallots, sliced
- 2 garlic cloves, crushed
- ½ bird's-eye chilli, deseeded & finely chopped
- 4 tbsp flat leaf parsley, chopped
- 400g/14oz ripe plum tomatoes, roughly chopped
- 800g/1¾oz tinned haricot beans, rinsed
- 600g/1lb 5oz peeled raw king prawns
- 2 tbsp lemon juice
- 125g/4oz red chicory/endive, shredded
- Lemon wedges to serve
- Salt & pepper to taste

Method

1 Gently sauté the shallots, garlic & chilli in the olive oil for a few minutes until softened.

2 Add the parsley, roughly chopped tomatoes & haricot beans and gently simmer for 15 minutes stirring occasionally.

3 Add the prawns & lemon juice and combine well. Cover and simmer for a further 10 minutes or until the prawns are cooked through.

4 Sprinkle with shredded chicory and serve with lemon wedges.

CHEF'S NOTE

If you prefer chicory cooked rather than raw just add it to the sauce a few minutes before the end of cooking.

CAPER VEG CIANFOTTA (V)

270 calories

Ingredients

- 3 tbsp olive oil
- 400g/14oz aubergines/eggplant, cubed
- 150g/5oz red onion, chopped
- 75g/3oz celery, chopped
- 2 garlic cloves, crushed
- 2 tbsp balsamic vinegar
- 2 tbsp capers, chopped

- 200g/7oz ripe tomatoes, roughly chopped
- 150g/5oz pitted olives, sliced
- 75g/3oz asparagus, chopped
- 150g/5oz purple sprouting broccoli, chopped
- 75g/3oz sultanas, roughly chopped
- 4 tbsp freshly chopped parsley
- Salt & pepper to taste

Method

1 Gently sauté the aubergines, onions, celery and garlic in the olive oil for a few minutes until softened.

2 Add the balsamic vinegar, capers, tomatoes, olives, asparagus, broccoli & sultanas and continue to cook for 20-25 minutes or until everything is cooked through and tender.

3 Sprinkle with chopped parsley and serve.

CHEF'S NOTE

This dish can also be served cold. Add a pinch of brown sugar if you feel the balance of flavour needs it.

CAPER & ANCHOVY TUNA SALAD

380 calories

Ingredients

- 1 medium free-range egg
- 75g/3oz ripe cherry tomatoes
- 125g /4oz tinned tuna steak, drained
- 6 anchovy fillets, drained and finely chopped
- 2 tsp capers, chopped
- 50g/2oz red onion, finely chopped
- 50g/2oz rocket leaves
- 50g/2oz baby kale leaves
- 1 tbsp extra virgin olive oil
- Lemon wedges to serve
- Salt & pepper to taste

Method

1 First place the egg in a saucepan and hard boil for about 5 minutes. When it's cooked, peel & leave to cool.

2 Meanwhile halve the cherry tomatoes and combine with the drained tuna steak, anchovies, chopped capers and red onion. Add the olive oil, seasoning & a squeeze of lemon and mix well.

3 Arrange the salad leaves and rocket onto a plate then sit the tuna & tomato mixture into the centre. Slice the egg in half lengthways and again into quarters.

4 Place the egg quarters on top of the salad and serve with lemon wedges.

CHEF'S NOTE
You could also make this simple salad with grilled fresh tuna.

WALNUT & ROASTED PEPPER SALAD (V)

390 calories

Ingredients

- 25g/1oz walnuts
- 50g/2oz red chicory/endive
- ½ cucumber
- 50g/2oz jarred roasted peppers, drained & chopped
- 1 tbsp balsamic vinegar
- 2 tsp lemon juice
- 1 tbsp extra virgin olive oil
- 2 tbsp freshly chopped mint
- 75g/3oz baby spinach leaves
- Salt & pepper to taste

Method

1 Finely slice the red chicory and use a vegetable peeler to peel the cucumber. Discard the cucumber skin and use the vegetable peeler to make cucumber ribbons. Use only the firm flesh, not the seeded core for this and discard the core when all the flesh is removed.

2 Mix together the sliced chicory, cucumber ribbons, peppers, balsamic vinegar, lemon juice, olive oil and mint. Season and toss with the spinach leaves. Sprinkle with the walnuts and serve.

CHEF'S NOTE
Walnuts contain powerful antioxidants.

BLUE CHEESE WATERCRESS OMELETTE (V)

520 calories

Ingredients

- 3 medium free-range eggs
- 50g/2oz stilton cheese, crumbled
- 2 tbsp freshly chopped flat leaf parsley
- 2 tsp extra virgin olive oil
- 50g/2oz red onion
- 50g/2oz watercress
- Salt & pepper to taste

Method

1 Lightly beat the eggs with a fork. Season well and add the crumbled stilton and parsley.

2 Gently heat the oil in a frying pan and sauté the red onion for a few minutes before tipping into the bowl with the beaten eggs. Pour the eggs and sautéed onion mixture back into the pan. Tilt the pan to ensure the mixture is evenly spread over the base.

3 Cook on a low to medium heat and, when the eggs are set underneath, fold the omelette in half and continue to cook for a few minutes.

4 Serve with the watercress on the side.

CHEF'S NOTE
Check the eggs are set underneath by lifting with a fork before folding the omelette in half.

QUICK TUNA & OLIVES

555 calories

Ingredients

- 2 tsp lemon juice
- 1 tbsp extra virgin olive oil
- 1 tsp balsamic vinegar
- 2 tsp Dijon mustard
- ½ garlic clove, crushed
- 50g/2oz red onion, sliced

- ½ red pepper, deseeded & sliced
- 50g/2oz vine ripened tomatoes, sliced
- 75g/3oz rocket
- 150g/5oz tinned tuna, drained
- 50g/2oz pitted black olives, sliced
- Salt & pepper to taste

Method

1 Make a dressing by mixing up the lemon, oil, vinegar, mustard & garlic with a good pinch of salt.

2 Load the onions, peppers, sliced tomatoes & rocket in a shallow bowl and use a fork to flake the tuna over the top.

3 Pour over the dressing and add the olives.

CHEF'S NOTE
A quick and easy lunch packed with omega oils.

QUINOA & CANNELLINI LUNCH BOX (V)

490 calories

Ingredients

- 100g/3½oz pre-cooked and cooled quinoa
- 1 garlic clove, crushed
- 1 tbsp red wine vinegar
- 1 tbsp olive oil
- 1-2 tsp lemon juice
- ½ birds eye chilli, deseeded & finely chopped
- Large pinch of salt

- 150g/5oz tinned cannellini beans, drained
- 1 baby gem lettuce
- 50g/2oz cherry tomatoes
- 50g/2oz red onion, chopped
- 75g/3oz tinned sweetcorn, drained
- 2 tbsp flat leaf parsley, chopped
- Salt & pepper to taste

Method

1 First make the dressing by mixing up the garlic, vinegar, olive oil, lemon juice, chillies and salt (alter the balance to suit your own taste).

2 Give the beans a quick rinse in cold water, dry them off and add to the same bowl as the dressing. Combine and put to one side.

3 Shred the lettuce, halve the cherry tomatoes and get them set up in a shallow bowl along with the chopped onion. Add the drained quinoa, tip the dressed beans over and pile the drained sweetcorn on top.

4 Sprinkle with flat leaf parsley, and store in an airtight lunchbox in the refrigerator.

CHEF'S NOTE
Pre cooked quinoa is readily available in pouches or just cook your own ahead of time to use in simple salad recipes.

CURRIED CAULIFLOWER & WALNUT SOUP (V)

245 calories

Ingredients

- 600g/1lb 5oz cauliflower florets
- 125g/4oz potatoes
- 1 tbsp extra virgin olive oil
- 75g/3oz shallots
- 1lt/4 cups vegetable stock/broth
- 1 tbsp medium curry powder
- 1 tsp turmeric
- 250ml/1 cup milk
- 50g/2oz walnuts, chopped
- 4 tbsp flat leaf parsley, chopped
- Salt & pepper to taste

Method

1 Quickly chop up the cauliflower & potatoes (no need to peel).

2 Heat the olive oil in a saucepan and add the shallots. Sauté for a minute or two before adding the stock, cauliflower, potatoes, turmeric & curry powder.

3 Turn up the heat, bring to the boil and simmer for 7-10 minutes or until all the vegetables are soft.

4 Add the milk, stir well and heat through for a minute.

5 Blend to a smooth consistency, check the seasoning and serve with the chopped walnuts and parsley sprinkled over the top.

CHEF'S NOTE
Add a little more stock if you want a thinner base to the soup.

THE *Skinny*
SIRT
food diet

PHASE ②
DINNER RECIPES
FOLLOW FOR 14 DAYS

SOYA BEAN & TOFU PENNE (V)

425 calories

Ingredients

- 200g/7oz tofu
- 300g/11oz buckwheat penne
- 1 tbsp extra virgin olive oil
- 1 garlic cloves, crushed
- 150g/5oz soya beans
- 150g/5oz fresh peas
- 120ml/½ cup low fat crème fraiche
- 2 tbsp freshly chopped mint
- Salt & pepper to taste

Method

1 First cube the tofu and dry off as much as possible.

2 Begin cooking the penne in a pan of boiling water until tender.

3 Meanwhile heat the olive oil in a high-sided frying pan and stir-fry the tofu for a few minutes on a high heat.

4 Reduce the heat, add the garlic, soya beans and peas and sauté for a few minutes. When the peas and beans are cooked through stir in the crème fraiche and mint.

5 Drain the cooked penne and add to the pan.

6 Toss well, season & serve with lots of freshly ground black pepper.

CHEF'S NOTE
The dryer the tofu is, the better it will stir-fry.

COCOA KHEEMA GHOTALA

480 calories

Ingredients

- 200g/7oz brown rice
- 2 tbsp extra virgin olive oil
- 50g/2oz red onion, sliced
- 1 garlic cloves, crushed
- 75g/3oz kale, finely sliced
- 75g/3oz beef tomatoes, roughly chopped
- 1 tbsp medium curry powder
- 1 tbsp cocoa powder
- 1 tsp ground turmeric
- 400g/14oz lean beef mince
- 4 medium free-range eggs
- 4 tbsp flat leaf parsley, chopped
- Salt & pepper to taste

Method

1 Place the rice in a pan of boiling water and cook until tender.

2 Meanwhile heat the oil in a frying pan and gently sauté the red onion & garlic for a few minutes until softened.

3 Add the kale, tomatoes, curry powder, cocoa powder, turmeric and mince to the pan. Increase the heat and brown for a few minutes.

4 Reduce the heat, stir well and cook for 6-10 minutes or until the mince is cooked through.

5 Whilst the rice is cooking break the eggs. Lightly beat with a fork and add to the mince. Stir though to scramble for a minute or two.

6 Add the drained rice and combine well. Season and serve with chopped parsley.

CHEF'S NOTE
For a spicy start to your day leave out the rice and serve this dish as a traditional Indian breakfast!

BROCCOLI & ANCHOVY FUSILLI

410 calories

Ingredients

- 300g/11oz buckwheat fusilli
- 8 tinned anchovy fillets
- 300g/11oz tenderstem broccoli/brocollini
- 3 tbsp extra virgin olive oil
- 2 garlic cloves, crushed
- 50g/2oz red onion, finely sliced
- 1 bird's-eye chilli, deseeded & finely chopped
- 75g/3oz spinach, chopped
- Salt & pepper to taste

Method

1 Cook the fusilli in a pan of boiling water until tender. Drain the anchovy fillets & roughly chop the tenderstem broccoli.

2 Heat the olive oil in a frying pan and gently sauté the garlic, red onion, chilli and chopped broccoli for a few minutes. Add the anchovy fillets and cook for a further 4-5 minutes until they begin to break up and the broccoli starts to become slightly tender (you still want it to retain a little crunch).

3 Drain the cooked pasta and add to the frying pan along with the chopped spinach. Combine for a minute or two, check the seasoning and serve.

CHEF'S NOTE
Tenderstem broccoli is great for making quick lunches and suppers. Try cooking the stems whole and serving with an anchovy, olive oil and chilli dressing.

PARSLEY PESTO SPAGHETTI (V)

584 calories

Ingredients

- 300g/11oz buckwheat noodles/spaghetti
- 75g/3oz shallots, sliced
- 4 servings parsley pesto (p102 for recipe)
- 75g/3oz watercress
- 25g/1oz Parmesan shavings
- Salt & pepper to taste

Method

1 Cook the buckwheat pasta in a pan of boiling water until tender.

2 Meanwhile heat the oil and gently sauté the shallots in a high-sided frying pan whilst the pasta cooks.

3 Drain the cooked pasta and add to the frying pan along with the parsley pesto. Toss well.

4 Sit the pasat on a bed of watercress, sprinkle Parmesan, season & serve.

CHEF'S NOTE
You could also use the Walnut pesto (p103 for recipe) this quick and easy Sirt supper.

SARDINE & FENNEL NOODLES

SERVES 4

590 calories

Ingredients

- 3 tbsp olive oil
- 100g/3½oz red onion, sliced
- 1 fennel bulb, finely chopped
- 2 garlic cloves, crushed
- 1 bird's-eye chilli, deseeded & finely chopped
- 300g/11oz fresh boneless sardine fillets, roughly chopped
- 75g/3oz medjool dates, finely chopped
- 2 tbsp water
- 2 tbsp tomato puree/paste
- 300g/11oz buckwheat noodles/spaghetti
- Lemon wedges to serve
- Salt & pepper to taste

Method

1 Heat the olive oil and gently sauté the onions, fennel, garlic & chillies for a few minutes until softened. Add the sardines, dates, water & tomato puree. Cover and leave to gently cook for 10-15 minutes. Meanwhile cook the pasta in a pan of boiling water until tender.

2 Check the sardines are cooked through and gently use a fork to mash and break up the fillets. Combine well. Add a little more water if you need to loosen it up.

3 Drain the pasta and combine everything really well. Season and serve with lemon wedges.

CHEF'S NOTE
You could use tinned sardines if you are short of time.

FRESH WALNUT & PARSLEY PASTA (V)

499 calories

Ingredients

- 300g/11oz buckwheat noodles/spaghetti
- 50g/2oz fresh walnuts
- 75g/3oz grated Parmesan cheese
- ½ tsp crushed sea salt
- 2 garlic cloves
- 6 tbsp flat leaf parsley
- 3 tbsp extra virgin olive oil
- 200g/7oz cherry tomatoes, finely chopped
- Salt & pepper to taste

Method

1 Cook the pasta in boiling water until tender. Meanwhile in a food processor place the walnuts, cheese, salt, garlic, parsley & olive oil and whizz into a paste.

2 Drain the pasta and place in a saucepan along with the walnut paste and fresh tomatoes. Combine well, warm through, season and serve.

CHEF'S NOTE
Walnuts and parsley combine to make a super Sirt sauce.

SOYA BEAN & PRAWN NOODLES

575 calories

Ingredients

- 1 tsp extra virgin olive oil
- ½ bird's-eye chilli, deseeded & finely chopped
- 1 garlic clove, crushed garlic
- 1 tsp grated fresh ginger
- 125g/4oz shelled king prawns
- 1 red pepper
- 2 tbsp soy sauce
- 75g/5oz soya beans
- 75g/3oz buckwheat noodles
- 1 bunch spring onions/scallions
- Salt & pepper to taste

Method

1 Heat the olive oil in a frying pan or wok and gently sauté the chilli, garlic and ginger for a minute or two. Add the prawns and cook for a few minutes until they begin to pink up.

2 Meanwhile quickly de-seed & slice the red pepper. Add to the pan along with the soya beans and soy sauce.

3 Stir-fry for 3-4 minutes whilst you cook the noodles in boiling water until tender.

4 Check the prawns are cooked through and when the noodles are ready, add to the pan. Combine for a minute or two.

5 Slice the spring onions and use these as a fresh garnish.

CHEF'S NOTE
Buckwheat is rich in Rutin which has anti-inflammatory properties.

BROCCOLI & ANCHOVY STIR-FRY

555 calories

Ingredients

- 6 tinned anchovy fillets
- 200g/7oz purple sprouting broccoli
- 1 tbsp extra virgin olive oil
- 1 garlic clove, crushed
- ½ bird's-eye chilli, deseeded & finely chopped
- 50g/2oz red onion, chopped
- 125g/4oz fresh tomotaoes, chopped
- 150g/5oz cooked brown rice (cooked weight)
- 2 tbsp chives, chopped
- Salt & pepper to taste

Method

1 Drain the anchovy fillets & roughly chop the broccoli.

2 Heat the olive oil in a frying pan or wok and gently sauté the garlic, red onion, tomatoes and chilli for 2 minutes. Add the anchovy fillets and cook for a further 2 minutes until they begin to break up.

3 Add the chopped broccoli to the pan

4 Stir-fry for 5-6 minutes whilst you microwave the rice.

5 When the rice is ready, check the broccoli is cooked to your liking, and add the rice to the pan.

6 Combine for a minute or two, check the seasoning and serve with the chopped chives on top.

CHEF'S NOTE
Sachets of cooked brown rice are readily available for quick lunches, or just cook a portion in the usual way.

FRESH HERB & TURMERIC PRAWNS

435 calories

Ingredients

- 1 tbsp extra virgin olive oil
- 1 garlic clove, crushed
- ½ bird's-eye chilli, deseeded & finely chopped
- 200g/7oz shelled, raw king prawns
- 1 tsp turmeric
- 1 tbsp soy sauce

- 1 tbsp Thai fish sauce
- 150g/5oz cooked brown rice (cooked weight)
- 1 tbsp freshly chopped coriander/cilantro
- 2 tbsp flat leaf parsley, chopped
- 1 bunch spring onions/scallions
- Salt & pepper to taste

Method

1 Heat the olive oil in a frying pan or wok and gently sauté the garlic and chillies for a minute or two.

2 Add the prawns, turmeric, soy sauce & fish sauce and cook until the prawns begin to pink up.

3 Check the prawns are cooked through, add the chopped herbs and rice to the pan. Combine for a minute or two.

4 Slice the spring onions and toss through the brown rice. Season & serve.

CHEF'S NOTE
This simple stir-fry contains 5 of the Top 20 Sirt foods.

CAULIFLOWER & HERB BROWN RISOTTO (V)

422 calories

Ingredients

- 3 tbsp olive oil
- 1 garlic clove, crushed
- 50g/2oz shallots, chopped
- 50g/2oz celery, finely chopped
- 300g/11oz wholemeal risotto
- 1lt/4 cups vegetable stock/broth
- 800g/1¾lb cauliflower
- ½ bird's-eye chilli, deseeded & finely chopped
- 4 tbsp freshly chopped chives
- 4 tbsp freshly chopped flat leaf parsley
- 50g/2oz rocket
- Salt & pepper to taste

Method

1 Heat the olive oil and gently sauté the shallots, celery and garlic for a few minutes until softened.

2 Add the risotto rice to the pan and stir well to coat each grain in olive oil. Add a ladle of stock and simmer until the stock is absorbed. Continue cooking the risotto adding a ladle of stock each time and allowing the rice to absorb the stock until adding the next ladle.

3 Continue cooking for about 15-20 minutes or until the rice is tender. Add more water or stock if needed.

4 Meanwhile quarter the cauliflower and place into a food processor. Pulse for a few seconds to make into rice size grains. Add to the risotto along with the sliced chillies. Combine well and continue cooking until the risotto rice and cauliflower 'rice' are both tender.

5 Add the chopped herbs, stir well, season and serve with the rocket on the side.

CHEF'S NOTE
You could also serve this with blanched kale rather than rocket.

ANCHOVY & OLIVE FAST STEW

420 calories

Ingredients

- 2 tbsp extra virgin olive oil
- 150g/5oz red onion, sliced
- 1 garlic clove, crushed
- 75g/3oz anchovy fillets, drained
- ½ bird's-eye chilli, deseeded & finely chopped
- 400g/14oz ripe plum tomatoes, roughly chopped
- 2 tbsp tomato puree/paste
- 120ml/½ cup red wine
- 150g/5oz pitted black olives, halved
- 2 tbsp lemon juice
- 800g/1¾lb skinless, boneless white fish filets
- 2 tbsp flat leaf parsley, chopped
- Salt & pepper to taste

Method

1 Preheat the oven to 200C/400F/Gas Mark 6.

2 Gently sauté the onion, garlic, anchovy fillets & chillies in the olive oil for a few minutes until softened.

3 Add the roughly chopped tomatoes, puree & wine and leave to gently simmer for 20 minutes stirring occasionally. Add the olives & lemon juice and combine well to make a rich tomato sauce.

4 Place the fish filets in an ovenproof dish and pour over the tomato sauce. Season well and place in the oven. Cook for 20-30 minutes or until the fish is cooked through and piping hot.

5 Sprinkle with chopped parsley and serve.

CHEF'S NOTE
The anchovy fillets give a lovely depth to this simple fish stew.

GRILLED TUNA & ROASTED KALE

417 calories

Ingredients

- 150g/5oz fresh tuna steak
- 1 tbsp extra virgin olive oil
- 125g/4oz kale, roughly chopped
- 1 tbsp red wine vinegar
- Large pinch sea salt flakes
- 1 tsp lemon juice
- 1 tbsp freshly chopped marjoram
- Lemon wedges to serve
- Salt & pepper to taste

Method

1 Preheat the oven to 160C/325f/Gas3

2 In a large bowl combine together the kale, vinegar, sea salt and olive oil. Arrange the kale in a single layer on a large baking tray and gently roast in the oven for 40 minutes.

3 After 30 minutes of cooking preheat the grill to a medium/high heat. Mix together lemon juice & marjoram and lightly brush on either side of the fish.

4 Place the tuna steak under the grill and cook for 2-3 minutes each side or until the tuna is cooked to your liking.

5 Arrange the cooked kale in a shallow bowl, Sit the tuna on top, and serve with lemon wedges on the side.

CHEF'S NOTE
Fresh tuna is best served rare in the centre, but feel free to adjust the cooking time to suit your own taste.

PARSLEY PESTO CHICKEN

594 calories

Ingredients

- 150g/5oz skinless chicken breasts
- 50g/2oz red onions, sliced into rounds
- 1 serving parsley pesto (p102 for recipe)
- 125g/4oz French beans
- 125g/4oz ripe cherry tomatoes, halved
- 2 tsp dried oregano
- 1 tbsp extra virgin olive oil
- Salt & pepper to taste

Method

1 Preheat the oven to 200/400/gas Mark 6

2 Hold the chicken breast as if you were slicing through the centre of it. Stop slicing before you cut it in half completely (butterfly the breast). Open the chicken breast to expose the two inside parts.

3 Spread the inside with the parsley pesto and close the 'sandwich' back up so you are left with pesto through the centre of the chicken breast.

4 Place the chicken, onions, beans and tomatoes in a casserole dish. Season well, sprinkle with the dried oregano and brush with olive oil.

5 Place in the oven and leave to cook for 30-40 minutes or until the chicken is cooked through and the vegetables are tender. Remove from the oven and arrange the beans, tomatoes and onions as a bed onto which you serve the chicken breast.

CHEF'S NOTE

Pesto is traditionally made with basil but using flat leaf parsley is great for your Sirt diet.

CANNELLINI BEAN SOUP (V)

440 calories

······ *Ingredients* ······

- 4 tbsp extra virgin olive oil
- 2 garlic cloves, crushed
- 75g/3oz celery
- 50g/2oz shallots, sliced
- 400g/14oz tinned cannellini beans

- 1.25lt/5 cups vegetable stock
- 200g/7oz whole wheat orzo pasta
- 4 servings walnut pesto (p103 for recipe)
- Salt & pepper to taste

······ *Method* ······

1 Heat the olive oil in a high-sided pan and gently sauté the garlic, celery & shallots, for a few minutes. Meanwhile cook the orzo in salted boiling water until tender, drain and put to one side.

2 Add the cannellini beans and stock to the onions, cover and leave to gently simmer for 20 minutes.

3 Remove two whole ladles of cannellini beans. Blend the rest of the beans and stock to a smooth consistency, add a little boiling water if needed. Combine together the cooked orzo, smooth sauce and reserved beans and divide into shallow bowls. Dollop a serving of walnut pesto in the middle of each bowl. Season & serve.

CHEF'S NOTE
If you are only cooking for one you can freeze the remaining portions.

CREAMY MUSHROOM & WALNUT SPAGHETTI (V)

440 calories

Ingredients

- 50g/2oz dried porcini mushrooms
- 300g/11oz buckwheat noodles/spaghetti
- 1 tbsp extra virgin olive oil
- 1 garlic clove, crushed
- 75g/3oz shallots, sliced
- 2 tsp dried thyme

- 2 tbsp mascarpone cheese
- 1 tbsp tomato puree/paste
- 50g/2oz walnuts pieces, chopped
- 4 tbsp flat leaf parsley, chopped
- Salt & pepper to taste

Method

1 Place the porcini mushrooms in a little boiling water and leave to rehydrate for 10-15 minutes. Thinly slice when softened.

2 Cook the spaghetti in a pan of boiling water until tender.

3 Heat the olive oil in a high-sided frying pan and gently sauté the garlic, shallots & dried thyme whilst the pasta cooks.

4 When the onions are soft add the mascarpone cheese and tomato puree & stir well. Drain the cooked pasta and add to the frying pan.

5 Toss well. Season & serve with the walnuts and parsley sprinkled over the top.

CHEF'S NOTE
Dried porcini mushrooms are readily available in any supermarket.

WALNUT CHICKEN CURRY

625 calories

Ingredients

- 300g/11oz brown rice
- 1 tbsp extra virgin olive oil
- 75g/3oz red onion, sliced
- 2 garlic cloves, crushed
- 400g/14oz vine ripened tomatoes, chopped
- 2 tsp turmeric
- 1 tbsp medium curry powder

- 500g/1lb 2oz chicken breast, cut into thick diagonal strips
- 1 tbsp coconut cream
- 2 tbsp flat leaf parsley, chopped
- 1 bird's-eye chilli, deseeded & very finely sliced
- 50g/2oz walnuts, chopped

Method

1 Cook the rice in a pan of boiling water until tender.

2 Heat the olive oil in a large non-stick frying pan or wok and sauté the red onions, and garlic for a few minutes until the onions begin to soften. Stir through the tomatoes, turmeric & curry powder and simmer for 5 minutes.

3 Add the chicken to the frying pan and simmer for 10-12 minutes or until the chicken is cooked through. Stir the coconut cream through the curry and divide over the rice.

4 Sprinkle with the fresh parsley, chillies and walnuts and serve.

CHEF'S NOTE
You could also make this simple curry with tofu rather than chicken.

LIME CHICKEN KEBAB

545 calories

Ingredients

- 75g/3oz quinoa
- 250ml/1 cup hot vegetable stock
- 1 garlic clove, crushed
- 1 tbsp extra virgin olive oil
- 2 tsp lime juice
- 125g/4oz skinless chicken breasts, cubed
- 50g/2oz baby spinach leaves
- 1 tbsp flat leaf parsley, chopped
- 1 tsp freshly chopped coriander/cilantro
- Salt & pepper to taste
- Metal skewers

Method

1 Put the quinoa and stock in a saucepan, cover and cook for about 20 minutes or until it's tender. (Add more stock if you need to and when it's ready drain off any excess liquid and put to one side).

2 Meanwhile preheat the grill to a medium/high heat.

3 Mix together the garlic, olive oil & lime juice in a bowl. Season the chicken and add to the bowl. Combine well and skewer each piece to make a large chicken kebab.

4 Place under the grill and cook for 6-8 minutes each side or until the chicken is cooked through and piping hot. Remove from the grill, and season.

5 Arrange the spinach and kebab on a plate, sprinkle with the chopped herbs and serve.

CHEF'S NOTE
This lovely meal can be made ahead and allowed to cool for a cold lunch.

THE *Skinny*
SIRT
food diet

SNACK & SAUCE
RECIPES

SWEET SOY EDAMAME (V)

207 calories

Ingredients

- 200g/7oz edamame (soya beans still in their pods)
- 1 tbsp honey

- 2 tbsp soy sauce
- 2 tbsp water
- 1 tsp extra virgin olive oil

Method

1 Add the edamame to a pan of boiling water and simmer for 4 minutes. Drain and pat dry.

2 Meanwhile heat a saucepan with the honey, soy sauce, water and oil. Simmer for a few minutes until the sauce begins to thicken slightly (make sure you don't burn the honey).

3 Toss the edamame in and combine well.

4 Delicious as a warm or cold snack.

CHEF'S NOTE
Try making a large batch of the sweet soy dressing so that you can make this easy snack anytime you like.

ROASTED GARLIC KALE CHIPS (V)

190 calories

Ingredients

- 200g/7oz kale
- 1-2 tsp sea salt flakes
- 2 tbsp extra virgin olive oil
- 1 garlic clove, crushed

Method

1 Preheat the oven to 180C/350F/Gas Mark 4.

2 Remove the thick stalks from the kale and tear the leaves into small bite size pieces.

3 Place these in a large bowl along with the salt, oil and garlic cloves.

4 Combine everything well and spread in a single layer on a baking sheet.

5 Bake in the oven for 12-15 minutes or until the edges begin to brown but are not burnt.

CHEF'S NOTE
This is a great snack to keep to hand throughout the day if you feel your energy levels dropping.

SERVES 1

SWEET NUT & SEED SNACK (V)

240 calories

Ingredients

- 75g/3oz pumpkin seeds
- 75g/3oz walnuts
- 1 tsp turmeric
- ½ tsp paprika
- 1 tsp sea salt flakes
- 1 tsp honey
- 1 tbsp extra virgin olive oil

Method

1 Preheat the oven to 180C/350F/Gas Mark 4.

2 Place all the ingredients into a large bowl and toss.

3 Combine everything really well and spread in a single layer on a baking sheet.

4 Bake in the oven for 12-15 minutes or until they are golden brown.

CHEF'S NOTE

Increase the honey if you like a particularly sweet snack.

CELERY & STRAWBERRY SNACK (V)

51 calories

Ingredients

- 1 celery stalk
- 1 tbsp cream cheese
- 4 strawberries

Method

1 Remove any green tops from the strawberries and very finely dice the strawberries.

2 Combine the strawberries with the cream cheese to make a paste.

3 Pile this along a celery stalk to create a simple Sirt snack you can eat immediately.

CHEF'S NOTE

You could make a large batch of strawberry cream cheese by blending it in a food processor to give it a smooth consistency.

PARSLEY PESTO (V)

204 calories

Ingredients

- 50g/2oz pine nuts
- 125g/5oz flat leaf parsley
- 50g/2oz Parmesan cheese
- 6 tbsp extra virgin olive oil
- 2 garlic cloves, crushed
- Salt & pepper

Method

1 Gently heat the pine nuts in a dry frying pan until golden. This will only take a minute or two, shake the pan occasionally.

2 Put all the ingredients into a food processor and pulse until smooth. Season and store for up to 5 days.

CHEF'S NOTE
Making pesto can be a question of personal choice. Adjust the balance of ingredients to suit your own taste.

WALNUT PESTO (V)

216 calories

Ingredients

- 50g/2oz walnuts
- 75g/3oz flat leaf parsley
- 75g/3oz Parmesan cheese
- 6 tbsp extra virgin olive oil
- 1 garlic clove, peeled
- Salt & pepper

Method

Put all the ingredients into a food processor and pulse until smooth. Season and store for up to 5 days.

CHEF'S NOTE
Using walnuts and parsley in this simple pesto is a great Sirt option you can use to add some excitement to many meals.

Other
COOKNATION
TITLES

If you enjoyed **The Skinny Sirtfood Diet Recipe Book** we'd really appreciate your feedback. Reviews help others decide if this is the right book for them so a moment of your time would be appreciated.

Thank you.

You may also be interested in other low calorie titles from CookNation. To browse our full catalogue visit **www.bellmackenzie.com**

Printed in Great Britain
by Amazon